The Parenting Advice

How to Use This Book

- Read the centre page of this book and remember it always. This is your parenting mantra!

- Record advice and thoughts on parenting that fit and makes sense for you, your child and family. Rip it out later if it no longer makes sense.

- Record precious moments and special things your child says or does. Add it to your child's baby albums later.

- Carry a crayon, pen, or marker wherever you go, and when your child is bored, bring it out so he/she can draw in this book, color, or play XXX's and OOO's with you.

- Tear the pages out to use as a grocery list.

Enjoy the journey!

BONUS GIFT! For an ebook download, free with purchase of this book, of "The Parenting Information Maze: An Overview of Parenting Philosophies, Styles and Programs," please email the ISBN number of this book to jarnall@shaw.ca

Arnall, Judy, 1960-
The last word on parenting advice / Judy Arnall.
ISBN 978-0-9780509-2-4
1. Parenting.
2. Child rearing.
I. Title. HQ769.A753 2011 649'.1 C2011-901090-9

Published by Professional Parenting Canada, Calgary, Alberta, Canada
jarnall@shaw.ca
www.professionalparenting.ca
Volume discounts available

First Edition 2011
Cover illustrations and design by:
PurpleWanda Creative, www.purplewanda.ca

Printed and bound in Canada

You are the best person in the world for your child.

Trust yourself.

You know what is right for you, your children and your family.

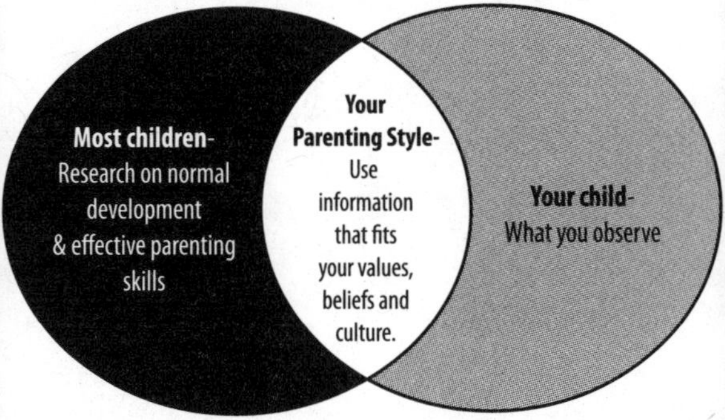

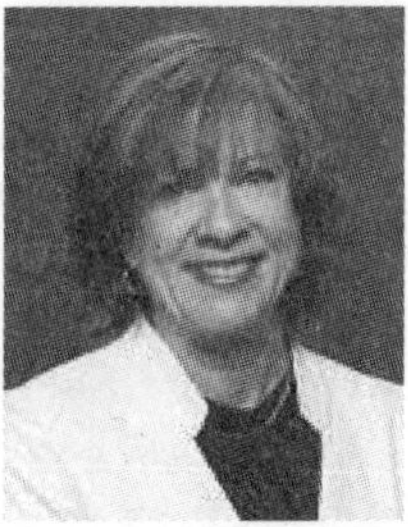

Judy Arnall

Parenting Speaker, Trainer and Bestselling Author
Judy is an international award-winning Toastmaster and CAPS professional speaker and Canadian parenting expert. She has given advice for television interviews on CBC, CTV, and Global as well as publications such as Chatelaine, Today's Parent, Canadian Living, Parents magazine and newspapers such as the Globe and Mail, Sun Media and Postmedia News. She teaches parenting at The University of Calgary, Continuing Education, Chinook Learning, and Alberta Health Services. Judy is the author of the bestseller, **Discipline Without Distress: 135 Tools for Raising Caring, Responsible Children Without Time-out, Spanking, Punishment or Bribery.** As a parent of five children, Judy has a broad understanding of the issues facing parents and the digital generation, and has just released an educational DVD titled **Plugged-In Parenting: Connecting with the Digital Generation for Health, Safety and Love.**

www.professionalparenting.ca
jarnall@shaw.ca **(403) 714-6766**

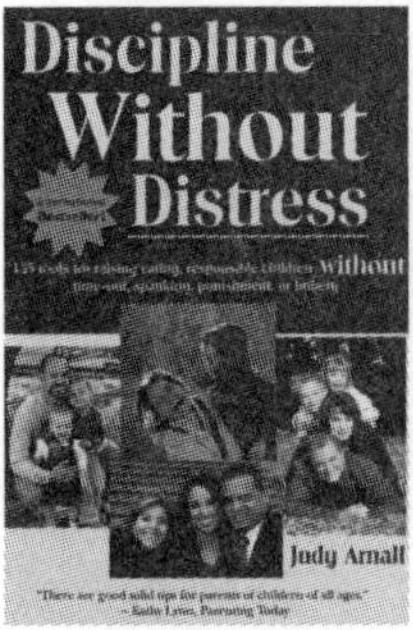

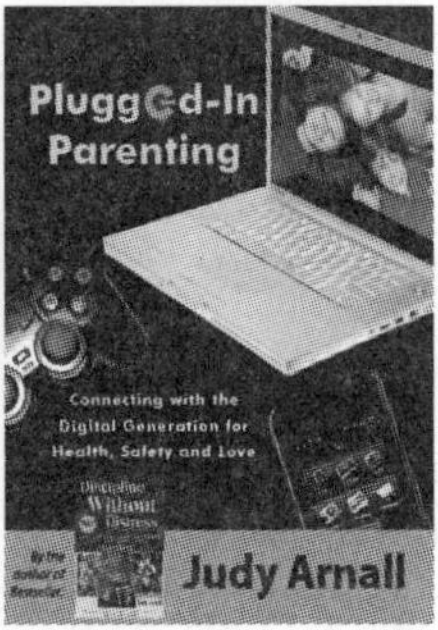